Table of Contents

INTRODUCTION

A balanced diet is key to maintaining a healthy weight and good health. It goes without saying that your body needs all the nutrients from foods to function correctly, such as carbohydrates, protein, fats, minerals, and vitamins. Therefore, a balanced diet contains foods of different varieties, quantities, and proportions to meet your body's nutritional requirements.While a balanced diet does not discriminate between food groups, you must have the right knowledge and guidance when eating "energy-rich but nutrient-poor" foods. There's no one-size-fits-all when it comes to a balanced diet. Since everyone has different nutritional needs, the right diet for good health varies from person to person. However, following a holistic diet that covers all the essential food groups and is low in unhealthy nutrients is an excellent way to live a healthy lifestyle.

WHAT IS A BALANCED DIET?

A balanced diet comprises the right proportion of foods from all the major food groups to provide the body with ideal nutrition. In general, it offers around 60-70% of total calories from complex carbohydrates, 20-25% of total calories from healthy fats, and 10-12% from proteins. However, these values differ based on individual requirement and various other factors.Following a healthy, balanced diet gives you enough energy, macronutrients, and micronutrients to stay healthy. The most important rule of balanced eating is to eat all meals without skipping any meal small or big. For a healthy average adult, a well-balanced diet typically includes three main meals and two snacks between meals. However, the food groups' proportion can be adjusted or modified based on your specific needs or health issues (if any).

A personalised balanced diet is vital since the bodily response to all foods is highly individual. Therefore, certain foods in one person's "good" diet can be part of another's "bad" diet. Instead of blindly following the universal dietary advice you see on the internet, HealthifyMe can help you with personal dietary recommendations after considering multiple factors.

With the help of these values and your other parameters, qualified dieticians customise your diet to match your body's needs and avoid potential adverse reactions to certain foods. The CGM device shows you how food affects your overall health in real-time and empowers you to make more informed decisions about your meal planning on a day-to-day basis. It unequivocally can lead to better long-term health outcomes.

Calories in a Balanced Diet

The ideal amount of calories in a balanced diet depends on whether you're trying to maintain the current weight, lose weight, or gain weight. If you want your weight to stay consistent, eat roughly the same amount of calories your body uses. The number of calories you need each day depends on many factors, such as age, gender, level of physical activity, and metabolism. For example, athletes who engage in high-intensity workouts require more calories than sedentary people. Similarly, pregnant women or adolescents going through a growth spurt need more calories than older adults. Therefore, a balanced diet that provides the right calories for your specific needs is crucial for overall fitness and well-being.

Why is a Balanced Diet Important?

The simple answer is eating a balanced diet helps you maintain good health and feel your best. While some people, such as athletes, may require additional dietary supplementation, most of us can get everything the body needs by eating various foods.In addition, studies show that the foods you eat profoundly impact your mental and physical health. So, your body becomes more vulnerable to chronic diseases, infection, and fatigue without balanced nutrition. Here is why nutritionally balanced diet is essential for every individual:

Helps Control Weight

Fad diets will come and go. A balanced diet is the only way to control and maintain your weight for the long term. A balanced diet may not result in weight loss as it does not focus on fat loss, rather it focuses on maintaining the current weight while giving appropriate nutrients for your body to function well.

Prevents Diseases and Infections

A balanced diet can safeguard you against chronic diseases such as diabetes, obesity, hypertension, and heart disease. In addition, the vitamins and minerals in a balanced diet build a robust immune system to fight infections.

Improves Your Mental Health

Some studies suggest a close relationship between diet and mental health. For example, a diet high in glycemic load may trigger depression and fatigue through hormonal imbalance. On the other hand, a balanced diet rich in vegetables, whole fruit, and whole grains improve the function of neurotransmitters and hormones, which enhances a good mood.

Maintain Brain Health

A study says that consistently following a balanced diet regime may protect us against cognitive decline and dementia. It is due to the appropriate amounts of vitamin D, vitamin C, vitamin E, and omega-3 fatty present in balanced diets. Getting the right mix of nutrients also promotes growth and better skin and hair.

What Makes Up a Healthy, Balanced Diet?
A balanced diet is a varied diet enriched with essential nutrients. However, eating a balanced diet can be simple. An excellent place to start is by incorporating five servings of fruits and vegetables into your daily routine. Here are the five major food groups you should include in your diet for optimum health:

Fruits and Vegetables

Fruit and vegetables are an integral part of any balanced diet. They are abundant in fibre, antioxidants, vitamins and minerals, essential for keeping the body healthy.

Fruit and vegetables should make up just over one-third of your daily diet, roughly five servings of different seasonal fruits and vegetables together per day. Let's take a peek at the colourful fruits and vegetables:

Red, orange, or yellow vegetables like tomatoes, bell peppers, carrots, sweet potatoes, and pumpkins are rich in lycopene, antioxidants beta carotene and vitamin C.

Purple and white vegetables like red cabbage, eggplant, cauliflower, mushrooms , berries, grapes rich in potassium, vitamin B, C and E.

Greens like spinach, brussels sprouts, beans, peas, and broccoli rich in vitamin A, C, K and, fibre.

Starchy Foods

Starchy foods or carbohydrates are the body's primary energy source, making up roughly one-third of your diet. Therefore, it is essential to understand the different types of starchy carbohydrates and choose healthier options to maintain a balanced diet. For example, replace processed foods with whole grains..

Choosing unrefined starchy carbs helps maintain digestive health and gives you more fibre, vitamins and minerals. Moreover, a study shows that whole grain consumption (rather than refined grains) reduces your risk of heart disease and type-2 diabetes.

Dairy

Dairy is the most well-known source of calcium and protein. For a balanced diet, go for low-fat or fat-free dairy options. Furthermore, eat fat-free flavoured yoghurts in moderation since they often contain added sugar.

If you are vegan, allergic, or intolerant to dairy, there are plant-based alternatives derived from soy, nut, oat, or rice. Also, choose fortified plant-based dairy to make up for the vitamins and minerals usually present in animal milk.

Protein

Protein, the storehouse of essential amino acids, must be one-eighth of your balanced diet. Protein rich foods not only help us in building muscles, but also boost our haemoglobin. Therefore, make sure to include varied protein sources.

It can be vegetarian sources such as beans, moong dal, urad dhal, paneer, tofu, nuts and seeds. For the non-vegetarians, good protein sources include eggs, oily fish and meat.While choosing meat, opt for lean cuts such as chicken and turkey and cut down on processed meats..

Healthy Fats

Fats are an essential part of a balanced diet and contribute to about 15-20% of daily caloric needs. They are also a significant energy source and help the body store and provide vitamins and synthesise hormones. However, it is essential to remember to use fats in moderation. While fat is an essential macronutrient, you need to be mindful of the type and amount of fat you consume. Always choose unsaturated fats over saturated fats. Saturated fats are present in red meat, pork, butter, margarine, cheese and coconut oil. Studies have shown that consuming too much of these foods can increase your heart disease and stroke risk. You can keep your heart healthy by choosing unsaturated fats from nuts, seeds, vegetable oils and fatty fish.

A balanced diet comprises foods from the five food groups: fruits and vegetables, starchy carbohydrates, protein, dairy and healthy fats. You are unlikely to include all five in every meal, so the aim is to achieve a healthy dietary balance across the day. This balance can be achieved by following a well planned balanced diet plan designed by a qualified nutritionist.In addition to solid foods, ensure that you drink at least 6-8 glasses of water daily since hydration is equally important.

FOODS TO EAT AND AVOID IN A BALANCED DIET

Foods to Eat

The vegetable group must include leafy greens, legumes or beans, starchy vegetables, and other colourful vegetables.

Nutritious protein choices include skinless poultry, lean beef and pork, fish, beans, peas, and legumes.

Eat low-fat dairy and soy products such as ricotta or cottage cheese, yoghurt, soy, or low-fat milk.

Healthful whole grains like brown rice, quinoa, oats, barley, and buckwheat

Fresh fruits, not juices, such as apples, berries, bananas, stone fruits, kiwi, melons, pomegranates, and other seasonal fruits you like

Foods to Avoid

Some of the food groups to avoid in a balanced diet include:

Processed foods

Refined grains

Alcohol

Added sugar and salt

Fatty cuts of red meat and processed meat

Trans and saturated fats

Packaged foods and beverages.

The plate method is an easy way to balance the food groups:

Half your plate with fruits and vegetables

Over one quarter with grains

Just under one quarter with protein

Adding dairy or a non-dairy replacement on the side

Sample Balanced Diet Charts for You to Try

Remember that the following plans are based on an average adult's standard weight and activity level. If you have any pre-existing medical conditions, make sure to follow the advice of your doctor or nutritionist.

A Balanced Vegetarian Diet Chart

With careful planning, a vegetarian diet can ensure daily requirements for nutrients such as calcium, iron, zinc, vitamin D, vitamin B12, healthy fats, and protein.

Day #1

Breakfast: Oatmeal bowl with fruit slices of your choice

Lunch: 1 cup of cooked brown rice with a bowl of dal, sabji and salad

Dinner: 1 cup rajma + 1 cup cucumber raita + 2 chapati

Snacks: 1 cup buttermilk + 5 almonds + 3 walnuts/ multigrain fat free khakra with tomato onion salad as a topping.

Day #2

Breakfast: 2 Idlis with vegetable sambar + green tea without sugar and milk

Lunch: low fatpaneer curry (3 pcs) + 2 roti or 1 bowl of rice+ salad

Dinner: 2 medium stuffed roti (vegetable/dal) + 1/2 bowl curd+ salad

Snacks: 1 cup watermelon + 5 almonds + dark chocolate (about six small pieces or two large squares)/ sprouts salad.

Day #3

Breakfast: 1 bowl of poha + 1 glass fruit yoghurt smoothie(without sugar)

Lunch: Stir-fried vegetables with brown rice + roasted tofu

Dinner: Stuffed eggplant + 1 cup cooked quinoa

Snacks: 1 glass buttermilk 1 cup chana chaat/ mixed vegetable tikki with curd dip.

Day #4

Breakfast: 2 besan chilla + 1 cup sprouts salad +

Lunch: Vegetable rice with one bowl of soya curry

Dinner: Homemade vegetable burger with baked sweet potato fries

Snacks: Steamed corn with black tea or coffee/ tossed green salad with cottage cheese/ sliced apple

Day #5

Breakfast: Upma with chutney + bowl of cut fruit.

Lunch: 2 chapatis with a bowl of soya chunks curry + sabji + salad or 1 bowl of vegetable khichdi + 1/2 cup yoghurt + sauteed soya chunks

Dinner: 1 cup quinoa with grilled veggies such as carrots, mushrooms, tomatoes, onions, broccoli and bell peppers

Snacks: Fruits salad/ Boiled chickpea salad

Day #6

Breakfast: A glass of lemon water + 2 Uttapam with coconut chutney

Lunch: A burrito bowl with brown rice, chickpea, salsa, flaxseeds, and other seasonings of your choice

Dinner: Bean soup with Greek yoghurt

Snacks: Brown bread sandwich with paneer filling/ Unsweetened fruit smoothie

Day #7

Breakfast: 2 medium-sized dosa with chutney + sambar

Lunch: 2 whole wheat chapatis + mixed vegetables curry + grilled mushrooms or paneer

Dinner: Mixed vegetable rice with bean sprouts salad + tossed soya chunks

Snacks: Tea with less sugar and milk + 2 digestive biscuits/ whole wheat toast + mixed fruits salad

A Balanced Non-Vegetarian Diet Chart

Day #1

Breakfast: Egg vegetable omelette (2 eggs) + 2 brown bread slices

Lunch: 2 roti + chicken curry with less oil + mixed vegetable salad

Dinner: 1/2 cup chana palak curry + 1/2 cup brown rice + cucumber carrot salad

Snacks: Tea/Coffee/Green Tea (1 Cup) + 4 almonds + 2 walnuts / Bowl of cut fruits

Day #2

Breakfast: 1 cup poha + 1 glass Tulsi tea + overnight soaked almond (5-6 pieces)

Lunch: A bowl of mixed vegetable rice + 1/2 cup of sprouted beans + 3-4 pieces of pan-seared chicken

Dinner: 2 roti + 1/2 cup dal (lentil/mung/chana)+ salad/sabji

Snacks: 2-3 wholegrain crackers with one slice of low-fat cheese/ crushed fruits slushie without sugar

Day #3

Breakfast: 1 glass low-fat milk + 2 boiled eggs + 2 pieces of multigrain/bread

Lunch: Roti/Rice + sabji + chicken (gravy/dry)

Dinner: 2 medium stuffed roti (vegetable/dal)+ 1 bowl of raita

Snacks: Frozen fruits (bananas, berries, or mangos) blended with peanut butter and Greek yoghurt

Day #4

Breakfast: Granola and fruit parfait

Lunch: Fish curry (2-3pcs) + rice (1 bowl)+ sabji or salad

Dinner: chicken sauteed (3 pcs) with mixed vegetable soup

Snacks: A banana drizzled with two teaspoons of melted dark chocolate

Day #5

Breakfast: Multigrain bread with peanut butter + 1 serving of seasonal fruit + 1 glass of milk

Lunch: Grilled salmon or mackerel + 1 cup brown rice + 1 cup any veg curry

Dinner: 1 cup of quinoa rice with grilled vegetables and baked sweet potato wedges

Snacks: 1 cup of fruit salad/ Chicken salad with bell pepper (1 quarter plate)

Day #6

Breakfast: 2 large eggs (poached or boiled) on whole grain toast with 1 tsp spread of choice + 1 cup of black coffee

Lunch: Whole grain pasta with a tomato-based sauce and chicken

Dinner: 2 tuna/chicken/turkey sandwiches

Snacks: A handful of nuts (30g) +1 cup of green tea/ bowl of mixed fruits with chia seeds and yogurt.

Day #7

Breakfast: Rolled oats with milk + fresh fruit

Lunch: Roasted vegetable, chicken & quinoa salad

Dinner: Grilled chicken (using olive oil) with mashed sweet potato and steamed vegetables

Snacks: 1 cup yoghurt topped with 1 tbsp mixed seeds/ sprouts chaat

A Balanced Vegan Diet Chart

Many people opt for vegan diet plans for various reasons, such as health, environmental or other personal preferences. A vegan diet excludes all animal products from the diet plan, including milk and milk products. Instead, it focuses on plant-based foods and beverages. It's essential to track your body's response when transitioning to a new diet, especially a vegan diet, to ensure you're getting the right mix of macro- and micronutrients.

Day #1

Breakfast: 1 cup sprouts salad + 2 stuffed paratha

Lunch: 1 cup vegetable fried rice + grilled soya chunks

Dinner: 2 tofu and vegetable sandwiches

Snacks: 1/2 cup roasted chickpeas + 1 glass of coconut water

Day #2

Breakfast: 1 cup steel-cut oats with veggies + 1 cup of almond milk

Lunch: 1 cup of bean salad + 1 cup quinoa buddha bowl

Dinner: 1 1/2 cups Moong dal khichdi + mixed vegetable salad

Snacks: 1 cup of edamame in pods or one medium apple

Day #3

Breakfast: 1 glass of strawberry pineapple smoothie + 1 bowl of overnight oats

Lunch: 2 chapati + 1/2 cup moong dal + sauteed mushrooms

Dinner: 1 cup of vegetable vermicelli + Boiled chana salad

Snacks: 1/2 cup of dry-roasted nuts and seeds of your choice

Day #4 .

Breakfast: Tea with dairy-free or plant-based milk + 2 idli/ uttapam with sambar

Lunch: 2 medium-sized vegetable wrap with mint chutney

Dinner: 2-3 stuffed besan cheela + vegan yogurt + salad

Snacks: 1 medium orange/ sprouts steamed

Day #5

Breakfast: 1 glass banana berries smoothie made with unsweetened soymilk + 2 vegan pancakes

Lunch: 2 avocado toast with fried tomatoes

Dinner: 2 cups mixed greens + 1/2 cup tofu stir fry + 1/2 cup rice

Snacks: 2 cups of air-popped popcorn/ sauteed boiled chana salad

Day #6

Breakfast: 2 slices of peanut butter and banana topping toast + 1 glass of lemon water/ besan cheela with mint chutney

Lunch: 1 cup quinoa + 1/2 cup chickpea curry/ brown rice with dal + sabji/salad

Dinner: 1/2 cup roasted cauliflower + 2 small whole-wheat bread slices + 1/3 cup hummus

Snacks: 1/2 cup of boiled corn and carrots + 1 cup of green tea

Day #7

Breakfast: 2 aloo paratha + mint coriander chutney + cup of mixed fruits

Lunch: 1 cup brown rice + 1 cup soy bean curry + 1/2 cup salad

Dinner: 2 chapatis + 1 cup mixed vegetable curry + sprouts salad

Snacks: 1/2 cup chana chaat + 1 cup black tea or black coffee

Dietary fat

Dietary fat contains more than double the kilojoules (energy) per gram than carbohydrate and protein. BAnimal products and some processed foods, especially fried fast food, are generally high in saturated fats, which have been linked to increased blood cholesterol levels. BReplacing foods high in saturated fats with alternatives higher in monounsaturated and polyunsaturated fats tends to improve blood cholesterol levels. It is important to select lower saturated fat varieties of core foods such as dairy products and meats. Following a Mediterranean diet, which is a diet high in healthy fats (such as extra virgin olive oil), fruits, vegetables, nuts, seeds, and whole grain breads and cereals, may reduce your risk of chronic disease development and increase your life expectancy. Foods and drinks contain nutrients (such as carbohydrates, proteins, fats, vitamins and minerals). Some foods or drinks contain a large amount of one nutrient such as soft drink, which contains a large amount of sugar, or fried food, which contains a large amount of fat.

The term 'fat' and 'oil' are often used to mean the same thing. Dietary fat (fat in foods and drinks) is important for many body processes. For example, it helps move some vitamins around the body and helps with making hormones. There are 4 types of dietary fat – each one can have a different effect on our blood cholesterol levels. For this reason, it is recommended to replace food and drinks high in saturated and trans fats with alternatives that contain more polyunsaturated or monounsaturated fats. Each gram of fat contains twice the kilojoules (energy) of carbohydrate or protein. Because of this, if you have foods and drinks with too much dietary fat, it can be difficult to maintain a healthy weight. Fats can bring out flavour in foods, so consuming meals with small amounts of fat can make foods more enjoyable and can satisfy our hunger for longer. Throughout the day you should consume a wide variety of foods including foods with small amounts of dietary fat, particularly polyunsaturated and monounsaturated fats, to meet your daily requirements.

Dietary fat has more than double the number of kilojoules per gram (37 kJ/g) than carbohydrate or protein (17 kJ/g), making it very 'energy dense'. Foods high in fat are usually high in kilojoules which means they are more likely to increase body fat. Therefore, it is recommended to choose 'low-fat' food options if the choice is available. Carrying too much body fat is a risk factor for many diseases, including cardiovascular disease, type 2 diabetes and many cancers.

Dietary fats and our blood cholesterol

The 2 types of blood cholesterol are low density lipoprotein (LDL) cholesterol and high-density lipoprotein (HDL) cholesterol. LDL is considered the 'bad' cholesterol because it contributes to the narrowing of the arteries, which can lead to cardiovascular diseases (such as heart disease and stroke). HDL cholesterol is considered 'good' cholesterol because it carries cholesterol from the blood back to the liver, where it is broken down – reducing the risk of cardiovascular disease.

Types of dietary fats
Dietary fat can be classified into 4 types. These are:

saturated

monounsaturated

polyunsaturated

trans.

Each type of fat behaves differently inside the body.

Saturated fats

Saturated fats (sometimes called 'bad fats') contribute to the risk of cardiovascular diseases (such as heart disease and stroke), because they raise our blood LDL cholesterol levels. These fats are commonly found in many discretionary foods and drinks (those to only have sometimes) – such as energy-dense takeaway ('fast food') meals and some commercial products (such as biscuits and pastries). Saturated fats are also found in some everyday, healthy foods (such as dairy products and meats). Unlike discretionary foods, these products have other important nutrients such as protein, vitamins and minerals, and can be important foods to include in your diet. It is recommended to select lower saturated fat options. For example, choose:

reduced-fat milk, yoghurt and cheese

leaner cuts of meat or trim the fat off meat prior to cooking.

Monounsaturated and polyunsaturated fats

Monounsaturated and polyunsaturated fats (sometimes called 'good fats') tend to lower your blood LDL cholesterol when they replace saturated fats in the diet.

Polyunsaturated fats have a slightly greater ability to reduce LDL cholesterol than monounsaturated fats.

Where possible, replace foods and drinks high in saturated fat with either monounsaturated or polyunsaturated alternatives. For example:

replace butter with olive oil or margarine

replace potato chips or chocolate with plain nuts as a healthier snack alternative

replace fried fast food with a sandwich or wrap made with lean meat and salad.

Limit trans fats

Trans fats tend to behave like saturated fats in the body, as they raise blood LDL cholesterol levels and increase the risk of cardiovascular diseases (such as heart disease and stroke). Unlike saturated fats, they tend to also lower HDL (good) cholesterol, so are likely to be even more damaging. Trans fats are rare in nature – they are only created in the stomach of cows and sheep. Because of this, trans fats are naturally found in small amounts in milk, cheese, beef and lamb. Trans fats can also be found in some processed foods (such as, pies, pastries, cakes, biscuits and buns) and in deep-fried takeaway meals. It is these trans fats produced during food manufacturing that we should be most concerned about, not the small amounts of trans fats naturally found in healthy foods like low-fat dairy products and lean meats.

Sources of dietary fat

Although foods can contain a mixture of different types of fat, they generally contain one main group of fat. Saturated fat sources include:

fatty cuts of meat

full-fat milk, cheese, butter, cream

most commercially baked products (such as biscuits and pastries)

most deep-fried fast foods

coconut and palm oil.

Monounsaturated fat sources include:

avocado, nuts (such as peanuts, hazelnuts, cashews and almonds – including peanut and other nut butters)

margarine spreads (such as canola or olive oil-based choices)

oils such as olive, canola and peanut.

Polyunsaturated fat sources include:

fish and seafood

polyunsaturated margarine

vegetable oils (such as safflower, sunflower, corn or soy oils)

nuts (such as walnuts and Brazil nuts) and seeds.

Plant sterols can lower cholesterol

Plant sterols are components in all plants that are very similar in structure to human cholesterol. Intakes of 2 to 3 g of plant sterols per day have been shown to reduce blood cholesterol levels by an average of 10%. This is because they block the body's ability to absorb cholesterol, which leads to a reduced level of cholesterol in the blood.

However, it is hard to eat this amount of plant sterols from natural sources, so there are now plant sterol-enriched margarine and dairy products on the market. Eating 1 to 1.5 tablespoons (4 to 6 teaspoons) of sterol-enriched margarine each day can help to lower blood cholesterol levels.

Fatty acids are essential in our diet

Fatty acids are a component of dietary fats that are necessary for vital functions in our bodies. There are 2 essential polyunsaturated fatty acids – omega-3 and omega-6. Essential means our bodies cannot create these fatty acids, so we must consume them in our diet. Omega-3 fatty acids are found in both plant and marine foods, although it is the omega-3 fatty acids from marine sources that have the strongest evidence for health benefits (including reducing the risk of heart disease). Plant food sources include canola and soy oils, canola-based margarine and seeds. Marine sources include fish, especially oily fish (such as Atlantic salmon, mackerel, Southern blue fin tuna, trevally and sardines). Omega-6 fatty acids are mainly found in nuts, seeds and plant oils (such as olive, corn, soy and safflower).

Benefits of omega-3 fatty acids
Research is ongoing, but the benefits of omega-3 fatty acids in the diet appear to be that they:

Lower the amount of fat in our blood and reduce blood pressure, (which are important risk factors in cardiovascular disease).

Improve blood vessel elasticity.

Keep the heart rhythm beating normally.

'Thin' the blood – which makes it less sticky and less likely to clot

Reduce inflammation and support the immune system.

May play a role in preventing and treating depression.

Contribute to the normal development of the foetal brain.

Olive oil

Olive oil is produced by the pressing or crushing of olive fruit. It comes in different grades, depending on the amount of processing involved. There are unrefined (virgin) grades and refined grades. The less the oil is refined by heat and chemical treatments, the higher the quality of the oil. Olive oil is an important source of omega-6 fatty acids and antioxidants, which are beneficial for overall health and can reduce risk of cardiovascular disease.

Types of olive oil
Virgin varieties of olive oil are believed to offer the greatest health benefits as they retain most of the healthy compounds from the olive fruit. Varieties include:

Extra virgin oil

Highest grade of oil from the first press of olives.

No chemicals and limited heat are used.

Most healthy compounds remain intact.

Virgin oil

Second best grade of oil from the second press of olives.

No chemicals and limited heat are used.

Most healthy compounds remain intact.

Olive oil

Lower quality oil that has been extracted from subsequent pressing of olives.

Some chemicals, heat and filters are used to refine the oil.

Small quantities of virgin olive oil are added to restore colour and flavour.

Light and extra light oil

Olive oil and the Mediterranean diet
Researchers are investigating the possibility that a diet rich in monounsaturated fats, (such as olive oil), may be protective against the development of coronary heart disease. People who have a high consumption of monounsaturated fats from olive oil (for example, in Greece and Italy) tend to have low rates of coronary heart disease, regardless of their body weight. Olive oil contains many compounds that are beneficial to human health, including omega-6 fatty acids, plant sterols and phenolic compounds, which seem to possess strong antioxidant properties. Because of these compounds, olive oil consumption may have a protective role against development of breast, colon, lung, ovarian and skin cancers.

Several studies have also shown that olive oil may have additional beneficial effects on blood pressure, obesity, rheumatoid arthritis and immune function. Recent research has also indicated a link between olive oil consumption as part of the Mediterranean diet, and reduced Alzheimer's disease risk. However, the Mediterranean diet contains much more than olive oil. It's possible that the low rate of coronary heart disease in these countries relates to a high intake of vegetables, legumes, fruits and cereals, which are all rich in antioxidants and plant sterols. Choosing extra virgin olive oil as your main source of dietary fat, as well as eating a healthy and balanced diet high in fruits, vegetables, nuts, seeds, and whole grain breads and cereals, may reduce your risk of chronic disease development and increase your life expectancy.

Balancing energy in and energy out

Achieving or maintaining a healthy weight is all about balancing the energy we take in with the energy we burn (energy out). Tips for watching the energy you take in:

- enjoy a variety of foods from each of the five food groups in the amounts recommended

- watch your portion sizes – particularly foods and drinks that are high in kilojoules

- limit your intake of energy-dense or high-kilojoule foods and drinks (check the kilojoules on the menu when eating out)

- if you do have an energy-dense meal, choose food or drinks that have fewer kilojoules at other meals in the day.

Tips for watching the energy you burn:

- be active in as many ways as you can throughout the day – take the stairs instead of the lift, get off the bus a stop early and walk, break up sitting time at work

- exercise regularly – at least 30 minutes of moderately intense activity on most days

- do more activity when you eat more kilojoules.

Achieving and maintaining a healthy weight is good for your overall vitality and well-being and helps prevent many diseases.

Energy in – eating too many kilojoules

When we regularly eat more kilojoules than our body needs, the spare energy is stored as fat. Eating as little as 100kJ extra each day (or burning 100kJ less by exercise), can lead to one kilogram of body fat creeping on over a single year. If you are above your healthy weight, to lose one kilogram (kg) of body fat in two months (without increasing your physical activity), you would need to eat around 600kJ less per day.

Energy in – eating too few kilojoules

When we regularly eat fewer kilojoules than our body needs our weight may decrease. If you experience weight loss that puts you outside of your healthy weight range or is unintentional, it is important to seek advice from your GP or Dietitian.

Energy out – exercise to burn kilojoules

When you are active, your body burns more energy (kilojoules). Exercise not only uses up stored energy, but also helps to stimulate muscle development. The more muscle tissue you have, the more kilojoules you can burn. Regular physical activity helps you manage your weight and maintain good health – it can even reduce your risk of chronic diseases. To actively lose weight, aim to do 60 – 90 minutes moderate-intensity physical activity most days of the week. Start small and gradually work your way up. Remember, weight you lose gradually is more likely to stay off than weight you lose through crash diets. If you are over 40, have a pre-existing medical condition or you haven't exercised for some time, see your doctor before starting a new fitness program.

Making practical changes to your energy balance

Reducing the amount of kilojoules we eat and drink every day, or doing more exercise every day, even by small amounts, can all add up and make a difference. This could be as easy as:

having salad or rice as a side instead of hot chips

ordering grilled instead of deep-fried or crumbed options

swapping full fat for low fat or skim milk

swapping a high sugar drink for water

swapping a fried food for a low kJ one

swapping a large food or drink serve for a smaller one

avoiding meal deal or 'two for one' promotions

checking the kilojoules on menus and choosing the lower kilojoule option

having fewer kilojoules at other meals

doing more activity when you eat more kilojoules.

HEALTHY EATING AND DIET

Eating a wide variety of healthy foods helps to keep you in good health and protects you against chronic disease. Eating a well-balanced diet means eating a variety of foods from each of the 5 food groups daily, in the recommended amounts. It is also important to choose a variety of foods from within each food group. Takeaway foods, cakes, biscuits and soft drinks are examples of foods usually high in saturated fat, added salt or added sugars. They should be considered as extras to your usual diet and only eaten occasionally and in small amounts.

Eat a variety of foods

Healthy eating means eating a wide variety of foods from each of the 5 major food groups, in the amounts recommended. Eating a variety of foods from the 5 major food groups provides a range of nutrients to the body, promotes good health and can help reduce the risk of disease - as well as keeping your diet interesting with different flavours and textures. Many of the foods that often feature regularly in modern diets do not form part of the 5 food groups. These foods, sometimes referred to as 'junk' foods, 'discretionary choices' or 'occasional foods' can be enjoyed sometimes, but should not feature regularly in a healthy diet. Fats and oils are high in kilojoules (energy) but necessary for a healthy diet in small amounts. No matter where you're starting, it's easy to make little changes to bring your eating closer in line with the Australian Dietary Guidelines. Just focus on eating foods from the 5 major food groups and reducing your intake of occasional foods.

5 major food groups

The Australian Guide to Healthy Eating groups the foods that should make up our daily diets into 5 major food groups. The 5 food groups are:

vegetables and legumes or beans

fruit

lean meats and poultry, fish, eggs, tofu, nuts and seeds, legumes or beans

grain (cereal) foods, mostly wholegrain or high cereal fibre varieties

milk, yoghurt, cheese or alternatives, mostly reduced fat.

Foods are grouped together because they provide similar amounts of key nutrients. For example, key nutrients of the milk, yoghurt, cheese and alternatives group include calcium and protein, while the fruit group is a good source of vitamins, especially vitamin C. Eating a varied, well-balanced diet means eating a variety of foods from each of the 5 food groups daily, in the recommended amounts. Because different foods provide different types and amounts of key nutrients, it is important to choose a variety of foods from within each food group. As a bonus, choosing a variety of foods will help to make your meals interesting, so that you don't get bored with your diet.

Occasional foods

Some foods do not fit into the 5 food groups because they are not necessary for a healthy diet. These foods are called 'discretionary choices' (sometimes referred to as 'junk foods') and they should only be eaten occasionally. They tend to be too high in saturated fat, added sugars, added salt or alcohol, and have low levels of important nutrients like fibre. These foods and drinks can also be too high in kilojoules (energy). Regularly eating more kilojoules than your body needs will lead to weight gain. Examples of 'discretionary choices' or occasional foods are:

sweet biscuits, cakes, desserts and pastries

processed meats and fatty, salty sausages, savoury pastries and pies, with a high fat or salt content

takeaway foods such as hot chips, hamburgers and pizza

sweetened condensed milk

alcoholic drinks

ice cream and other ice confections

confectionary and chocolate

commercially fried foods

potato chips, crisps and other fatty and/or salty snack foods including some savoury biscuits

cream, butter and spreads which are high in saturated fats

sugar-sweetened soft drinks and cordials, sports and energy drinks.

It's okay to have some of these foods now and then as an extra treat. But if these foods regularly replace more nutritious and healthier foods in your diet, your risk of developing obesity and chronic disease, such as heart disease, stroke, type 2 diabetes, and some forms of cancer, increases.

Restaurant meals and takeaway foods

Restaurant meals and takeaway foods are often high in saturated fat, added salt, added sugars, and kilojoules. Think about how often you consume food and drinks prepared outside the home. If you're doing this regularly, consider cutting back and focusing more on the 5 major food groups. That doesn't mean you have to stop completely. Suggestions for reducing saturated fat in takeaway food options include:

Try ordering a takeaway meal without the fries.

Choose bread-based options like wraps, kebabs, souvlaki or hamburgers.

Avoid deep fried and pastry options.

Include extra vegetables and salad.

Choose smaller portions or share with someone else and add a green salad to reduce the kilojoules of the meal.

Limit high fat, high salt sauces and toppings like cheese, fatty meats and mayonnaise – remember, you can ask for less.

Choose tomato-based pasta sauces, rather than cream-based sauces.

Drink plenty of water.

Don't upsize unless it's with a side salad.

Fast foods that have relatively low levels of saturated fat and added salt include:

pizzas with less cheese and meat

grilled chicken burgers or wraps

grilled, lean meat hamburgers, with no cheese or bacon additions

grilled fish burgers.

High sugar foods

Foods and drinks like soft drinks, cordials, biscuits, cakes and confectionary are high in added sugars and high in kilojoules. Sugar itself does not lead to diabetes. But added sugars can cause weight gain and being overweight increases a person's risk of type 2 diabetes. Sugar-sweetened drinks are the largest source of sugars in the diets of Australians. There is strong evidence of an association between increasing consumption of sugar-sweetened drinks and the development of childhood obesity and tooth decay. That's why eating foods and drinks with a high sugar content should be limited. Sugar-free versions are okay to drink sometimes, but sugar-free fizzy drinks are still acidic, which can have a negative effect on bone and dental health. Water is the healthiest drink – try adding a slice of lemon, lime or orange for flavour.

High-salt foods

Too much salt in the diet has been associated with an increased risk of high blood pressure, which is a known risk factor for heart disease and stroke. Eating less than 5 g of salt per day (less than a teaspoon a day) is recommended for adults with normal blood pressure. Many Australians consume double this amount each day. The majority of our salt intake comes from packaged and processed foods we eat every day, like bread, processed meats and soups. Cutting back on takeaway foods will help reduce your salt intake.

Healthy fats
The Australian Dietary Guidelines include a small allowance for healthy fats each day (around one to 2 tablespoons for adults and less for children). Consuming unsaturated (healthy) fats in small amounts is an important part of a healthy diet. It helps with:

the absorption of vitamins (A, D, E and K)

reducing your risk of heart disease

lowering your cholesterol levels - if the healthy fats replace saturated (bad) fats in your diet.

There are 2 main types of unsaturated fats:

monounsaturated fats - found in olive and canola oil, avocados, cashews and almonds

polyunsaturated fats, such as:

omega-3 fats - found in oily fish

omega-6 fats - found in safflower and soybean oil, and Brazil nuts.

The best way to include healthy fats in your diet is to replace saturated fat that you may currently be eating (such as butter and cream) with a healthier, unsaturated fat option (such as olive oil or a polyunsaturated margarine).

How much do I need from each food group each day?
How much you need from each food group each day depends on your age, gender and activity levels. The Australian Guide to Healthy Eating outlines how many serves you and your family need each day, and standard serve sizes for foods and drinks.

Daily serves needed by children and teenagers

Children and adolescents

Grain (cereal) foods, mostly wholegrain

Vegetables and legumes or beans

Fruit

Milk, yoghurt, cheese or alternatives (mostly reduced fat)

Lean meat and poultry, fish, eggs, nuts and seeds, legumes or beans

Toddlers 1-2 years*

4

2-3

½

1-1½

1

Children 2-3 years

4

2½

1

1½

1

Children 4-8 years

4

4½

1½

2 (boys),1½ (girls)

1½

Children 9-11 years

5 for boys

4 for girls

5

2

2 ½ for boys

3 for girls

2 ½

Adolescents 12-13 years

6 for boys

5 for girls

5 ½ for boys

5 for girls

2

3 ½

2 ½

Adolescents 14-18 years

7

5 ½ for boys

5 for girls

2

3 ½

2 ½

Pregnant and breastfeeding girls under 18 years

8

5

2

3½

3½

Breastfeeding girls under 18 years

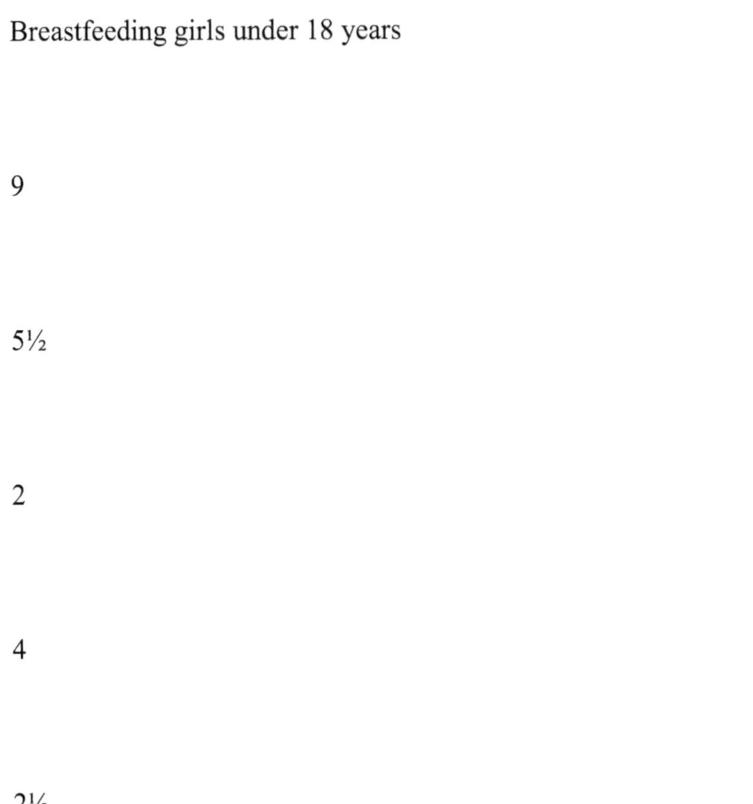

9

5½

2

4

2½

*An extra serve (7-10 g) per day of unsaturated spreads or oils or nut or seed paste is included as whole nuts and seeds are not recommended for children of this age due to potential choking risks.

Daily serves needed by women

Women

Grain (cereal) foods, mostly wholegrain

Vegetables and legumes or beans

Fruit

Milk, yoghurt, cheese or alternatives (mostly reduced fat)

Lean meat and poultry, fish, eggs, nuts and seeds, legumes or beans

19-50 years

6

5

2

2 ½

2 ½

51-70 years

4

5

2

4

2

Pregnant

8 ½

5

2

2 ½

3 ½

Breastfeeding

9

7 ½

2

2 ½

2 ½

70+ years

3

5

2

4

2

Daily serves needed by men

Men

Grain (cereal) foods, mostly wholegrain

Vegetables and legumes or beans

Fruit

Milk, yoghurt, cheese or alternatives (mostly reduced fat)

Lean meat and poultry, fish, eggs, nuts and seeds, legumes or beans

19-50 years

6

6

2

2 ½

3

51-70

6

5 ½

2

2 ½

2 ½

70+ years

4 ½

5

2

3 ½

2 ½

What counts as a daily food serve?

Standard serve sizes vary according to the type of food and the food group.

Vegetables - daily serve

One standard serve of vegetables is about 75 g (100 to 350 kJ) or:

½ cup cooked vegetables (for example, broccoli, carrots, spinach or pumpkin)

½ cup cooked dried or canned beans, peas or lentils (preferably with no added salt)

1 cup of green leafy or raw salad vegetables

½ cup sweet corn

½ medium potato or other starchy vegetables (such as sweet potato)

1 medium tomato.

Fruit - daily serve

One standard serve of fruit is about 150 g (350 kJ) or:

1 medium piece (for example, apple, banana, orange, pear)

2 small pieces (for example, apricots, plums, kiwi fruit)

1 cup diced or canned fruit (no added sugar).

Only occasionally, one standard serve of fruit can be:

125 ml (½ cup) fruit juice (no added sugar)

30 g dried fruit (for example, 4 dried apricot halves, 1½ tablespoons of sultanas).

Grain (cereal) foods - daily serve

Choose mostly wholegrain or high cereal fibre varieties of grain foods.

One standard serve is (500 kJ) or:

1 slice (40 g) of bread

½ medium roll (40 g) or flatbread

½ cup (75-120 g) cooked rice, pasta, noodles, barley, buckwheat, semolina, polenta, bulgur or quinoa

½ cup (120 g) cooked porridge

¼ cup (30 g) muesli

2/3 cup (30 g) breakfast cereal flakes

3 (35g) crispbreads

1 crumpet (60 g)

1 small (35 g) English muffin or scone.

Lean meats and poultry, fish, eggs, tofu, nuts and seeds and legumes/beans - daily serve

One standard serve is (500 to 600 kJ):

65 g cooked lean red meat such as beef, lamb, veal, pork, goat or kangaroo (about 90 to 100 g raw)

80 g cooked poultry such as chicken or turkey (100 g raw)

100 g cooked fish fillet (about 115 g raw weight) or 1 small can of fish

2 large (120 g) eggs

1 cup (150 g) cooked dried or canned legumes/beans such as lentils, chick peas or split peas (preferably with no added salt)

170 g tofu

30 g nuts, seeds, peanut or almond butter or tahini or other nut or seed paste (no added salt)*.

*Only to be used occasionally as a substitute for other foods in the group.

Milk, yoghurt, cheese and/or alternatives - daily serve

Milk, yoghurt and cheese should mostly be reduced fat.

One standard serve (500-600 kJ) is:

1 cup (250 ml) fresh, UHT long-life, reconstituted powdered milk or buttermilk

½ cup (120 ml) evaporated milk

2 slices (40 g) or one 4 x 3 x 2 cm cube (40 g) of hard cheese, such as cheddar

½ cup (120 g) ricotta cheese

¾ cup (200 g) yoghurt

1 cup (250 ml) soy, rice or other cereal drink with at least 100 mg of added calcium per 100 ml.

If you do not eat any foods from this group, the following foods contain about the same amount of calcium as a serve of milk, yoghurt, cheese or alternatives:

100 g almonds with skin

60 g sardines, canned, in water

½ cup (100 g) canned pink salmon with bones

100 g firm tofu (check the label - calcium levels vary).

Be mindful that some of these contain more kilojoules (energy), especially the nuts.

Change the way you think about food

There are lots of myths about healthy food. Don't make food choices based on false beliefs. Some things to try include:

Don't think that your diet must be 'all or nothing'. Eating well doesn't mean you must worry about eating healthily all the time. A good diet allows for treats occasionally.

Compare the prices of junk foods against the price of healthier food options to see that 'healthy' doesn't have to mean 'expensive'.

Experiment with different foods and recipes. A meal cooked with fresh ingredients is better than a limp burger or soggy chips.

Try different 'fast' options like whole-wheat breakfast cereal, muesli, wholemeal bread, wholegrain muffins, fruit, yoghurt or pasta.

When eating out, look for kilojoule labelling on menus and check before you choose. A single energy-dense meal may contain most of an adult's daily kilojoule intake, and drinks can be high in kilojoules too.

Don't give up your favourite meals entirely. Try thinking of new ways to create healthy meals – for example, you could make recipes lower in fat by changing the cooking method – grill, stir-fry, bake, boil or microwave, instead of deep frying.

Reduce the size of your meal or food instead of giving it up entirely. More doesn't always mean better.

If you're worried about missing out on socialising, instead of meeting friends for food, perhaps go for a walk instead. Or you could suggest a food outlet that serves healthier foods, such as wholemeal rolls with vegetable fillings, or sushi.

Get organised with food planning

Planning ahead can make changing your dietary habits a whole lot easier:

Make a shopping list before you shop and plan what meals you're going to eat and when.

Keep a filled fruit bowl at home for fast, low-kilojoule snacks.

Vary your meals. You may get bored and lose motivation if you don't try different ingredients and recipes.

Search the internet to find interesting and easy recipes and cooking tips – have a read of these tasty recipes.

Cook in bulk to save time – for example, soups, stews, casseroles and bolognese sauce are all easy to cook a lot of, and then freeze in portions for later use.

Eat breakfast every day so you're less likely to snack on occasional foods at morning tea. A wholemeal or wholegrain breakfast cereal that is low in sugar, served with low-fat milk, can provide plenty of vitamins, minerals and fibre. Other fast and healthy options include yoghurt or wholemeal toast.

Stock your food cupboard and fridge
Stock your food cupboard and fridge with ingredients that are quick to prepare and easy to cook. suggestions include:

Soups – easy to make and nutritious, especially if you add lots of vegetables, beans or lentils. You can use canned tomatoes and ready-made (low salt) stock as a base and add your own herbs, spices and leftovers.

Pasta – quick and easy to prepare. Keep tins of tomatoes in your cupboard and add your own variations and flavours.

Rice – try making fried rice or risotto, or mix cooked rice with leftover vegetables and meat.

Beans and lentils – canned varieties can make a quick and nutritious addition to soups and stews. Lentils and beans can be used as a main meal with vegetables added.

Vegetables and fruit – make vegetable curries, stir-fries and vegetable patties and soups. Canned and frozen vegetables can easily be added to last minute meals. Fruit is good for a quick nutritious snack.

Meat and fish – tinned tuna is a great cupboard stand-by. Shop for cheap cuts of meat for slow cooking in stews and casseroles.

Condiments – add flavour and interest to your cooking. Keep a selection of dried herbs, spices, curry powder, vinegars, in your cupboard. Tomato sauce, soy sauce and stock cubes also provide great flavour, but they are high in salt – use them only in small amounts.

Healthy eating on a budget

Healthy doesn't mean expensive. Here are some ways to save money on food:

Cook extra for the evening meal so you can use the leftovers for a quick meal the following night or for lunch.

Cook double the amount then freeze what is left over in meal-size portions.

Shop at the local markets close to closing time for discounted fruit, vegetable and meat bargains.

Buy in bulk (it's usually cheaper) and freeze in smaller portion sizes to use as required.

Use cheaper cuts of meat for curries and casseroles for long slow cooking, then add extra vegetables and beans to make the meal go further.

One-pot dishes where you throw everything in together save energy, time, money and washing up.

Watch out for supermarket specials of staples (rice, pasta, pasta sauces, bread and tinned vegetables) and stock up on them when they are cheap. Bread can be frozen for at least two months, and items such as pasta and rice have a long shelf life.

Limit takeaway foods – they can be expensive, high in fat, high in salt, low in nutrition, and leave you hungry again a few hours after you eat them.

Buy fresh produce in season – it's often cheaper as it's grown locally and fresher.

COOKING TIPS FOR BUSY PEOPLE

There are many reasons why people are cooking less often. People's lives are busier; the two-income household can mean that neither partner has the time or energy to cook every night. There are also more people living alone, who often don't want to cook for themselves. However, convenience foods can be expensive and many are high in fat and salt. Fast foods are up to 65% higher in kilojoules and larger in portion size than food prepared at home. The average fast-food meal contains about half the kilojoules needed for the day, so many people are eating far too many kilojoules without realising it. If you lack the time or motivation to cook, the following suggestions may be helpful.

Keep your pantry well stocked

You may be tempted to order takeaway if your pantry is bare and you can't face the thought of going to the supermarket. The secret is to stock long-life ingredients that can be combined in any number of ways to create interesting dishes. Suggestions include:

Buy long-lasting vegetables like potatoes, pumpkins, carrots and onions, which can form the basis of soups or casseroles.

Keep tins of legumes on hand (for example, lentils, kidney beans, three-bean mix, chickpeas).

Stock a range of canned fish – for variety, include tuna, salmon and sardines.

Use tinned tomatoes, tomato paste, tinned corn or other tinned vegetables (look for 'no added salt' varieties) for pasta sauces, soups or casseroles.

Keep a selection of other long-life carbohydrates like rice (stock different varieties such as white, brown, arborio and jasmine), Asian-type dry noodles, and couscous.

Stock plenty of dried pasta, such as spaghetti, fettuccine, macaroni and spiral varieties.

Keep a supply of canned soups in the pantry (look for 'no added salt' varieties).

Have a stock of oils and vinegars, including olive oil, sesame oil, balsamic vinegar and red wine vinegar. You can make a wide range of salad dressings or marinades with these ingredients if you include a dash of herbs and lemon juice.

Stock dried herbs, including basil, coriander, mint, thyme, oregano and mixed herbs.

Useful condiments include tomato sauce, mustard, mayonnaise, relish, stock cubes, curry powder, ready-made stock, soy sauce and chilli sauce.

Store a variety of nuts – these are a great meat alternative, and can be added to salads, stir-fries or pasta dishes.

Make the most of your freezer and fridge

Keep your fridge and freezer stocked with handy, healthy food. For example:

Buy frozen vegetables and fruits (eg berries, mango). Contrary to popular belief, frozen fruit and vegetables retain a high proportion of their nutrients.

Crushed garlic and ginger are available in jars and fresh herbs are available in tubes to keep in the fridge.

Apples, pears and citrus fruits (eg oranges) have a long life when refrigerated.

Fresh lemon and lime juice can be bought in bottles and stored in the fridge.

Keep a supply of eggs in the fridge. Eggs are a versatile ingredient for a quick, easy and healthy meal.

Marinated tofu keeps well in the fridge and is easy to toss through a stir-fry with a few vegetables.

Grated cheese can be sealed and stored in the freezer to increase its shelf life.

When buying fresh meat, choose de-boned varieties. Divide the quantities into meal-sized portions and freeze separately.

Buy red meat and chicken already sliced or diced or marinated.

Buy bread in bulk and keep it in the freezer until needed.

Meal suggestions for busy people

The above pantry and fridge items can offer you a range of easily prepared main meals including:

stir fries

salads

curries

soups

casseroles

stews

pasta

risottos

Time-saving cooking suggestions for busy people

Suggestions include:

Make your time in the kitchen count - make double (or even quadruple) the quantity you need. Freeze the remainder in meal portions, and you have ready-made meals for later in the week or month.

Double up on tasks – you can save time if you do 2 things at once. For example, prepare your pasta sauce while your spaghetti is cooking.

Prepare one-pot meals – such as soups, risottos, slow-cooked curries and casseroles to save on time and washing up.

Use a microwave – it's easier and quicker to microwave foods than cook them in the oven or on the stovetop. Check your manufacturer's instructions on how to best cook different foods using your microwave.

Don't throw out leftovers – store them appropriately (such as refrigerating or freezing) for a quick meal the next day. Or reinvent the leftovers in a creative way; for example, pasta sauce can make a tasty jaffle filling.

Do some meal prep the night before and put the slow cooker on whilst you're at work, or have ingredients ready to make a quick meal when you arrive home.

Find your motivation for cooking

Some people who live alone don't like to cook for themselves. Different ways to motivate yourself include:

Invite people over for dinner more often.

Offer to go round to a friend's house to cook for them one night (hopefully, they will then return the favour one night for you).

If you have a child in your life (such as a grandchild, niece or nephew), involve them in cooking sessions. Most children enjoy preparing and cooking food, and you can have a lot of fun together

If your problem is coming up with interesting meals, a good cookbook can inspire you, or browse the web for easy, quick-to-prepare recipe ideas. Some food packets also have easy recipes on them.

Think of the money you'll be saving by cooking, instead of eating convenience foods (and how much better it is for you). Use the saved money to buy yourself a treat.

Healthy cooking tips and recipe suggestions

Eating a wide variety of healthy foods helps to keep you in good health and protects you against chronic disease. Eating a well-balanced diet means eating a variety of foods from each of the 5 food groups daily, in the recommended amounts. Find out more in the Australian Guide to Healthy Eating. Eating healthy food doesn't mean giving up your favourite recipes. Some simple swaps and a little bit of planning can help you make life-long, healthy changes to your diet.

Shop for healthy food
Some shopping tips to get you started:

Make a shopping list before you shop and plan what meals you're going to eat.

Keep the pantry stocked with ingredients that are quick to prepare and easy to cook.

Stock up on seasonal vegetables, fruit, wholegrains, nuts and seeds.

Choose the lower fat versions of a food if possible – for example milk, cheese, yoghurt, salad dressings and gravies.

Choose lean meat cuts and skinless chicken breasts.

Limit fast foods, chips, crisps, processed meats, pastries and pies, which all contain large amounts of fat.

Switch to healthier fats

Choose lean meats and reduced-fat dairy products and limit processed foods to minimise hidden fats. Nuts, seeds, fish, soy, olives and avocado are all healthier options because they include the essential long-chain fatty acids and these fats are accompanied by other good nutrients. If you add fats when cooking, use healthier oils such as olive and canola oil. And try these tips to reduce the amount of fat needed in cooking:

Cook in liquids (such as stock, wine, lemon juice, fruit juice, vinegar or water) instead of oil.

Use pesto, salsas, chutneys and vinegars in place of sour creams, butter and creamy sauces.

Use reduced fat yoghurt and milks, evaporated skim milk or corn-starch instead of cream in sauces or soups.

Use non-stick cookware to reduce the need for cooking oil.

When browning vegetables, put them in a hot pan then spray with oil, rather than adding the oil first to the pan. This reduces the amount of oil that vegetables absorb during cooking.

As an alternative to browning vegetables by pan-frying, it is good to cook them first in the microwave, then crisp them under the grill for a minute or 2.

Retain the nutrients

Water-soluble vitamins are delicate and easily destroyed during preparation and cooking. To minimise nutrient losses:

Scrub vegetables rather than peel them, as many nutrients are found close to the skin.

Microwave or steam vegetables instead of boiling them.

When boiling vegetables, use a small amount of water and do not overboil them.

Include more stir-fry recipes in your diet. Stir-fried vegetables are cooked quickly to retain their crunch (and associated nutrients).Reduce salt

Salt is hidden in many of our foods, but a high salt diet can contribute to a range of health problems including high blood pressure. Suggestions to reduce salt include:

Don't automatically add salt to your food – taste it first.

Add a splash of olive oil, vinegar or lemon juice close to the end of cooking time or to cooked vegetables – it can enhance flavours in the same way as salt.

Choose fresh or frozen vegetables, since canned and pickled vegetables tend to be packaged with salt.

Limit your consumption of salty processed meats such as salami, ham, corned beef, bacon, smoked salmon, frankfurters and chicken loaf.

Iodised salt is best. A major dietary source of iodine is plant foods. Yet there is evidence that Australian soil may be low in iodine and so plants grown in it are also low in iodine. If you eat fish at least once a week, the need for iodised salt is reduced.

Avoid processed foods such as flavoured instant pasta or noodles, canned or dehydrated soup mixes, salty crackers, chips and salted nuts.

Reduce your use of soy sauce, tomato sauce and processed sauces, stock powders and condiments (for example mayonnaise and salad dressings) because they contain high levels of salt.

Add flavour with herbs and spices
Herbs and spices can be used to add delicious flavours without the need for salt or oil. Here are a few tips you can try:

Fresh herbs are delicately flavoured so add them to your cooking in the last few minutes.

Dried herbs are more strongly flavoured than fresh. As a general rule, one teaspoon of dried herbs equals 4 teaspoons of fresh.

Add herbs and spices to soups, breads, mustards, salad dressings, vinegars, desserts and drinks.

Try some coriander, ginger, garlic, chilli and lemongrass with vegetables for a quick, healthy and delicious stir-fry.

Sandwich suggestions

For delicious healthy sandwiches:

Switch to wholemeal or wholegrain bread.

Include extra vegetables and salad fillings wherever possible

Replace butter with avocado, nut spreads, hummus or margarine spreads made from canola, sunflower or olive oils.

Choose reduced fat cheese or mayonnaise wherever you can.

Instead of processed meats, try alternatives like lean chicken, felafel, canned tuna or salmon.

Enjoy toasted sandwiches with baked beans.

Other things to keep in mind

Additional suggestions for healthy eating include:

Take time out to enjoy eating, away from screens and other distractions, and eat with others when you can.

You are less likely to overeat if you eat slowly and savour every mouthful.

And remember small changes, big impact. Making small, gradual changes to your diet (rather than restrictive eating or crash diets) will help you adopt healthy eating habits for life.